PLANT-BASED DIET FOR AUTOIMMUNE DISEASE

Optimize Health And Manage Symptoms With Nutrient-Rich Plant Based-Nutrition

Charlotte Harry

Table of Contents

CHAPTER ONE 5

INTRODUCTION TO AUTOIMMUNE DISEASES 5

DEFINITION AND OVERVIEW 9

COMMON AUTOIMMUNE DISEASES 14

SYMPTOMS AND DIAGNOSIS 17

CURRENT TREATMENT APPROACHES 20

CHAPTER TWO 24

THE ROLE OF DIET IN AUTOIMMUNE DISEASES 24

HISTORICAL PERSPECTIVES 28

SCIENTIFIC EVIDENCE LINKING DIET AND AUTOIMMUNE
CONDITIONS 31

WHY DIET MATTERS: INFLAMMATION AND IMMUNE
RESPONSE 34

CHAPTER THREE..38

UNDERSTANDING PLANT-BASED DIETS 38

WHAT CONSTITUTES A PLANT-BASED DIET? 42

TYPES OF PLANT-BASED DIETS.......................................45

NUTRITIONAL BENEFITS OF A PLANT-BASED DIET.............48

CHAPTER FOUR 53

PLANT-BASED DIETS AND INFLAMMATION 53

HOW PLANT-BASED DIETS REDUCE INFLAMMATION...........56

KEY ANTI-INFLAMMATORY NUTRIENTS IN PLANT FOODS.....60

CASE STUDIES AND RESEARCH FINDINGS 64

CHAPTER FIVE 69

ESSENTIAL NUTRIENTS IN A PLANT-BASED DIET 69

MACRONUTRIENTS: PROTEIN, CARBOHYDRATES, FATS 73

MICRONUTRIENTS: VITAMINS AND MINERALS 75

SOURCES OF ESSENTIAL NUTRIENTS IN PLANT-BASED FOODS 79

CHAPTER SIX 83

PLANNING A BALANCED PLANT-BASED DIET FOR AUTOIMMUNE HEALTH 83

MEAL PLANNING AND PREPARATION...................................88

BALANCING MACRONUTRIENTS AND MICRONUTRIENTS 92

TIPS FOR ENSURING ADEQUATE PROTEIN AND OTHER KEY NUTRIENTS...95

CHAPTER SEVEN 101

SUPERFOODS AND SUPPLEMENTS FOR AUTOIMMUNE SUPPORT 101

TOP ANTI-INFLAMMATORY SUPERFOODS...........................107

SUPPLEMENTS TO CONSIDER 112

HERBAL REMEDIES AND THEIR BENEFITS 115

CHAPTER EIGHT 121

PRACTICAL TIPS FOR TRANSITIONING TO A PLANT-BASED DIET 121

GRADUAL TRANSITION STRATEGIES 124

OVERCOMING COMMON CHALLENGES 128

TIPS FOR EATING OUT AND SOCIAL SITUATIONS.................131

CHAPTER NINE 135

MANAGING SPECIFIC AUTOIMMUNE DISEASES WITH A PLANT-BASED DIET...135

CHAPTER TEN...156

RECIPES AND MEAL PLANS.................................156

BREAKFAST, LUNCH, AND DINNER RECIPES.......................159

SNACK AND SMOOTHIE IDEAS.............................163

SAMPLE WEEKLY MEAL PLAN.............................166

THE END...173

CHAPTER ONE

INTRODUCTION TO AUTOIMMUNE DISEASES

Autoimmune diseases are a group of disorders where the body's immune system mistakenly attacks its own tissues and organs. Normally, the immune system protects the body from harmful invaders like bacteria and viruses. In autoimmune diseases, this system gets confused and targets healthy cells, causing various symptoms and health problems.

There are over 80 different types of autoimmune diseases, each affecting different parts of the body. Some common examples include rheumatoid arthritis, where the immune system attacks the joints; type 1 diabetes, which targets insulin-producing cells in the pancreas; and multiple sclerosis, where the immune system damages the protective covering of nerve cells.

The exact cause of autoimmune diseases is not fully understood, but a combination of genetic, environmental, and lifestyle factors are believed to play a role. Genetics can make some people more prone to developing these conditions. For example, if a family member has an autoimmune disease, you might have a higher risk of getting one too. Environmental factors like infections, exposure to certain chemicals, and even diet may also trigger autoimmune responses in susceptible individuals.

Symptoms of autoimmune diseases can vary widely depending on the specific condition and the part of the body affected. Common symptoms include fatigue, joint pain and swelling, skin problems, abdominal pain, recurring fever, and swollen glands. Because these symptoms can be similar to those of other diseases, diagnosing an autoimmune disease can be challenging and often involves a combination of blood tests, imaging studies, and physical examinations.

Treatment for autoimmune diseases focuses on reducing inflammation, controlling symptoms, and preventing further damage to the body. This can involve medications such as nonsteroidal anti-inflammatory drugs (NSAIDs), corticosteroids, and immunosuppressive drugs that dampen the immune response. Lifestyle changes, such as a healthy diet, regular exercise, and stress management, can also help manage symptoms and improve quality of life.

Living with an autoimmune disease can be difficult, but many people manage their conditions successfully with proper medical care and support. It's important for individuals with autoimmune diseases to work closely with their healthcare providers to develop a personalized treatment plan. Additionally, support groups and counseling can provide emotional support and practical advice for coping with the daily challenges of these chronic conditions.

Autoimmune diseases are complex and can affect anyone, causing the immune system to attack the body's own tissues. While the causes are not entirely clear, understanding the symptoms and getting appropriate treatment can help individuals lead active and fulfilling lives despite their condition.

DEFINITION AND OVERVIEW

Autoimmune diseases represent a complex category of disorders wherein the body's immune system, typically tasked with defending against external threats such as bacteria and viruses, mistakenly attacks its own healthy tissues. This phenomenon arises from a malfunction where the immune system fails to differentiate between foreign invaders and the body's own cells and tissues, leading to a cascade of inflammatory responses and tissue damage.

The immune system functions through a sophisticated network of cells, tissues, and organs designed to identify and neutralize harmful substances. Central to this defense are antibodies and specialized cells that target and eliminate pathogens. In autoimmune diseases, however, this finely tuned system becomes disrupted. Normally, immune cells undergo rigorous screening processes to ensure they recognize and respond only to foreign antigens. This self-tolerance prevents the immune system from attacking the body's own cells, maintaining a delicate balance between protection and potential harm.

When this self-tolerance breaks down, immune cells start to produce autoantibodies—antibodies that target the body's own tissues—or T cells that mistakenly attack healthy cells. This aberrant immune response triggers inflammation and can damage various organs and tissues depending on the specific autoimmune condition. The exact cause of this breakdown in self-tolerance is not fully understood, but it is believed to involve a combination of genetic predisposition and environmental factors.

There are over 80 recognized autoimmune diseases, each with unique characteristics and targets within the body. Examples include rheumatoid arthritis, lupus, multiple sclerosis, type 1 diabetes, and Hashimoto's thyroiditis, among others. Symptoms vary widely depending on which tissues or organs are affected and can range from mild to severe. Common symptoms include fatigue, joint pain, rash, fever, and general malaise, which can significantly impact a person's quality of life.

Diagnosing autoimmune diseases can be challenging due to their diverse symptoms and the overlap with other conditions. Doctors typically rely on a combination of patient history, physical examination, blood tests to detect autoantibodies, and imaging studies to assess the extent of tissue damage. Treatment strategies often focus on managing symptoms, reducing inflammation, and suppressing the immune response to minimize tissue damage. Medications such as corticosteroids, immunosuppressants, and biologics are commonly used depending on the severity and specific characteristics of the autoimmune disease.

Research into autoimmune diseases continues to evolve, with ongoing efforts to understand their underlying mechanisms and develop more targeted therapies. This field of study holds promise for improved diagnostic methods, personalized treatment approaches, and ultimately, better outcomes for individuals affected by these challenging conditions.

COMMON AUTOIMMUNE DISEASES

One of the most prevalent autoimmune diseases is Rheumatoid Arthritis (RA), primarily impacting joints by causing inflammation, stiffness, and swelling. Another significant condition is Lupus, which can affect various organs such as the skin, joints, kidneys, and heart, leading to inflammation and tissue damage in these areas.

Multiple Sclerosis (MS) targets the central nervous system, resulting in nerve damage that manifests as symptoms like numbness, weakness, and debilitating fatigue. Type 1 Diabetes arises from the immune system's assault on insulin-producing cells in the pancreas, necessitating lifelong management of blood sugar levels.

Hashimoto's Thyroiditis represents an autoimmune attack on the thyroid gland, resulting in hypothyroidism and its associated symptoms like fatigue, weight gain, and sensitivity to cold. Inflammatory Bowel Disease (IBD), encompassing conditions like Crohn's disease and ulcerative colitis, involves chronic inflammation of the gastrointestinal tract, leading to symptoms such as abdominal pain, diarrhea, and weight loss.

Psoriasis, characterized by rapid skin cell turnover, causes patches of thickened, red skin covered with silvery scales. This autoimmune skin disorder can significantly impact quality of life due to its visible and often uncomfortable symptoms.

The severity of autoimmune diseases varies widely; while some individuals may experience mild discomfort or manageable symptoms, others face chronic pain, disability, and even life-threatening complications. Treatment strategies typically focus on alleviating symptoms, suppressing immune system activity, and managing any associated organ damage or dysfunction.

SYMPTOMS AND DIAGNOSIS

Autoimmune diseases encompass a spectrum of conditions where the immune system mistakenly attacks the body's own tissues. Symptoms can vary widely depending on the specific disease and the organs involved. Common manifestations include persistent fatigue, joint pain accompanied by swelling, muscle weakness, skin rashes or ulcers, recurrent fevers, cognitive difficulties such as trouble concentrating or memory lapses, digestive disturbances, and hair loss.

Diagnosing autoimmune diseases presents a challenge due to their diverse symptoms, which often overlap with those of other illnesses. To navigate this complexity, healthcare providers employ a multifaceted approach. This typically begins with a thorough medical history and comprehensive physical examination to identify any signs indicative of autoimmune activity. Blood tests play a crucial role by detecting specific antibodies that the immune system produces against its own tissues, as well as markers of inflammation which are often elevated in autoimmune conditions.

In addition to blood work, imaging studies like X-rays, CT scans, or MRIs may be utilized to visualize affected organs or tissues and assess the extent of damage. In certain cases, a biopsy of the affected tissue may be necessary to confirm the diagnosis definitively. This involves extracting a small sample of tissue for microscopic examination to observe characteristic abnormalities or immune cell infiltration.

Given the complexity and variability of autoimmune diseases, accurate diagnosis relies on a combination of clinical expertise and a systematic approach to interpreting symptoms and test results. Early detection is crucial for implementing timely treatment strategies aimed at managing symptoms, preventing organ damage, and improving overall quality of life for individuals affected by these often chronic and unpredictable conditions.

CURRENT TREATMENT APPROACHES

Current treatment approaches for autoimmune diseases primarily aim to alleviate symptoms, manage inflammation, and prevent organ damage since there is no known cure for most of these conditions. These strategies encompass a variety of medical interventions, lifestyle adjustments, physical therapies, and complementary treatments.

Medications play a central role in autoimmune disease management. Nonsteroidal anti-inflammatory drugs (NSAIDs) are commonly used to reduce pain and inflammation. Corticosteroids are potent anti-inflammatory agents that help control immune responses. Disease-modifying antirheumatic drugs (DMARDs) and biologic therapies target specific components of the immune system to suppress abnormal immune activity and prevent further tissue damage.

Lifestyle changes are pivotal in managing autoimmune diseases. Regular exercise can improve overall health, reduce inflammation, and enhance mobility. Stress management techniques such as meditation, yoga, and counseling can help mitigate stress-induced exacerbations of symptoms. Dietary modifications, often focusing on anti-inflammatory foods and sometimes elimination diets, aim to support immune function and reduce inflammation.

Physical therapy is frequently employed to improve joint mobility, muscle strength, and overall physical function in individuals with autoimmune diseases. It helps manage pain and prevents disability by tailoring exercises and techniques to the specific needs and limitations of each patient.

In addition to conventional treatments, many individuals explore alternative therapies to complement their medical regimens. Practices like acupuncture and massage therapy are believed to alleviate pain and promote relaxation,

potentially offering relief from symptoms. Herbal supplements are also utilized by some patients, although their efficacy and safety can vary widely and should be approached with caution.

Overall, managing autoimmune diseases involves a multifaceted approach that integrates medical interventions, lifestyle adjustments, physical therapies, and, in some cases, complementary treatments. The goal is to achieve symptom control, reduce inflammation, and maintain or improve quality of life for individuals living with these chronic conditions.

CHAPTER TWO

THE ROLE OF DIET IN AUTOIMMUNE DISEASES

Diet plays a crucial role in managing autoimmune diseases, influencing both their development and their symptoms. Autoimmune diseases occur when the immune system mistakenly attacks healthy cells in the body. While genetics play a significant role in their onset, environmental factors such as diet can either exacerbate or mitigate the immune response.

One key aspect of diet in autoimmune diseases is inflammation. Many autoimmune conditions, like rheumatoid arthritis, lupus, and Crohn's disease, are characterized by chronic inflammation. Certain foods, such as processed sugars, refined carbohydrates, and saturated fats, can promote inflammation in the body. In contrast, a diet rich in fruits, vegetables, whole grains, and healthy fats (like those found in nuts and fish) can help reduce inflammation and potentially alleviate symptoms.

Another important consideration is gut health. The gut houses a large portion of the body's immune system, and its microbial balance plays a critical role in immune function. Some studies suggest that an imbalance in gut bacteria, known as dysbiosis, may contribute to the development or exacerbation of autoimmune diseases. A diet high in fiber, probiotics (found in fermented foods like yogurt and kimchi), and prebiotics (found in foods like garlic, onions, and bananas) can support a healthy gut microbiome and potentially reduce autoimmune symptoms.

Moreover, certain foods may trigger autoimmune flare-ups in susceptible individuals. These triggers can vary widely between individuals, but common culprits include gluten, dairy, and nightshade vegetables (like tomatoes, peppers, and eggplants). Keeping a food diary or undergoing an elimination diet under the guidance of a healthcare professional can help identify specific triggers and allow for personalized dietary adjustments.

Vitamin and mineral deficiencies are also common in autoimmune diseases due to factors such as malabsorption or increased nutrient needs. For example, vitamin D deficiency is often seen in autoimmune conditions and has been linked to disease severity. Incorporating foods rich in essential nutrients, or taking supplements as recommended by a healthcare provider, can help support overall health and immune function.

It's important to note that while diet can play a significant role in managing autoimmune diseases, it is typically not a substitute for medical treatment. Individuals with autoimmune conditions should work closely with healthcare professionals to develop a comprehensive treatment plan that may include medications, lifestyle modifications, and dietary changes tailored to their specific needs.

HISTORICAL PERSPECTIVES

Throughout history, the concept that diet can impact health has persisted across civilizations. Ancient societies acknowledged the therapeutic potential of specific foods and herbs, although their knowledge primarily stemmed from empirical observations rather than rigorous scientific validation. These early beliefs laid the groundwork for understanding the interplay between diet and health.

In more contemporary eras, anecdotal accounts and limited studies hinted at the possibility that dietary modifications might alleviate symptoms associated with certain autoimmune disorders. These tentative findings spurred interest but lacked substantial scientific substantiation until the latter part of the 20th century.

The late 20th century marked a pivotal shift as scientific inquiry delved deeper into the connection between diet and health outcomes. Researchers began to systematically investigate how dietary patterns could influence various aspects of health, including autoimmune conditions. This era saw the emergence of controlled studies and clinical trials designed to elucidate the mechanisms underlying these effects.

Advancements in technology and research methodologies enabled scientists to explore complex interactions between diet, immune function, and disease processes. Gradually, a clearer picture began to emerge, highlighting specific dietary components that could either exacerbate or mitigate autoimmune symptoms. These insights represented a significant departure from earlier anecdotal evidence, providing a more robust foundation for understanding the therapeutic potential of diet in managing autoimmune conditions.

However, while ancient civilizations recognized the healing properties of food based on empirical knowledge, it wasn't until modern scientific inquiry gained momentum in the late 20th century that the profound impact of diet on health, particularly in autoimmune contexts, began to be systematically studied and understood. This evolution underscores the ongoing exploration and validation of the age-old concept that what we eat can profoundly influence our well-being.

SCIENTIFIC EVIDENCE LINKING DIET AND AUTOIMMUNE CONDITIONS

Scientific research over recent decades has extensively explored the relationship between diet and autoimmune diseases, uncovering several significant insights:

Firstly, dietary patterns rich in fruits, vegetables, whole grains, and healthy fats (like those in olive oil and nuts) have consistently shown associations with lower inflammation levels. Inflammation, a hallmark of autoimmune conditions, contributes to tissue damage and symptom severity.

Secondly, the gut microbiota, comprising trillions of microbes, critically influence immune system regulation. Diets high in fiber and plant-based foods promote a diverse gut microbiota, potentially modulating immune responses and reducing autoimmune activity.

Certain diets have demonstrated promise in managing autoimmune diseases, though they are not cures. For example, the Mediterranean Diet, abundant in fruits, vegetables, whole grains, fish, and olive oil, is linked to reduced inflammation and improved cardiovascular health, beneficial for autoimmune patients. Similarly, the Anti-Inflammatory Diet emphasizes foods like omega-3 fatty acids (found in fish and flaxseeds), turmeric, ginger, and leafy greens to combat inflammation. Additionally, Elimination Diets, supervised medically, involve temporarily excluding potential trigger foods (such as gluten or dairy) to assess symptom improvement.

Nutrients such as vitamin D, vitamin A, omega-3 fatty acids, and antioxidants (abundant in colorful fruits and vegetables) are crucial for immune function and may help regulate autoimmune responses.

WHY DIET MATTERS: INFLAMMATION AND IMMUNE RESPONSE

Diet plays a pivotal role in autoimmune diseases due to its profound influence on inflammation and immune system function. In autoimmune conditions, chronic inflammation is a significant driver of tissue damage and symptom severity. Certain dietary components, such as saturated fats, refined sugars, and processed foods, have been shown to exacerbate inflammation. These foods can activate inflammatory pathways in the body, contributing to the persistent inflammatory state characteristic of autoimmune diseases.

Conversely, adopting a diet rich in anti-inflammatory components can help mitigate these effects. Antioxidants found in fruits, vegetables, and whole grains possess anti-inflammatory properties that can counteract oxidative stress and inflammation. Similarly, omega-3 fatty acids found in fatty fish, flaxseeds, and walnuts have been shown to reduce inflammation by modulating immune responses and decreasing pro-inflammatory cytokines.

The immune system's functionality is also profoundly influenced by dietary choices. Nutrient deficiencies or imbalances can impair immune responses, potentially triggering or exacerbating autoimmune reactions. For example, deficiencies in vitamin D, vitamin A, zinc, and selenium have been linked to compromised immune function. Ensuring adequate intake of these nutrients through a balanced diet or supplementation may help support immune health and regulate autoimmune responses.

Furthermore, the gut microbiota and intestinal barrier integrity play crucial roles in immune system modulation. A diet high in fiber, prebiotics, and probiotics promotes a diverse and healthy gut microbiome. This microbial diversity is associated with improved immune function and reduced inflammation. In contrast, diets low in fiber and high in processed foods can disrupt the gut microbiota, leading to increased intestinal permeability (leaky gut) and heightened immune activation, which may exacerbate autoimmune symptoms.

CHAPTER THREE

UNDERSTANDING PLANT-BASED DIETS

Plant-based diets focus primarily on foods derived from plants, including fruits, vegetables, grains, nuts, seeds, and legumes, with little to no animal products. The emphasis is on whole, unprocessed foods that offer a range of nutrients vital for health.

One of the main reasons people choose plant-based diets is for their health benefits. Such diets are typically rich in fiber, vitamins, and minerals while being lower in saturated fats and cholesterol compared to diets that include meat and dairy. This composition can contribute to lower risks of heart disease, high blood pressure, and type 2 diabetes.

Another key aspect of plant-based diets is their environmental impact. Producing plant foods generally requires fewer resources, such as water and land, compared to raising animals for meat. Additionally, plant-based diets tend to generate fewer greenhouse gases and contribute less to environmental degradation, making them more sustainable choices for those concerned about the planet.

Ethical considerations also play a significant role for many people adopting plant-based diets. Avoiding animal products can align with concerns about animal welfare and the ethics of industrial farming practices. By opting for plant foods, individuals often feel they are reducing harm to animals and promoting more compassionate choices.

Variety is crucial in a plant-based diet to ensure all essential nutrients are obtained. This includes consuming a diverse array of fruits, vegetables, whole grains, nuts, seeds, and legumes. These foods provide different vitamins, minerals, and antioxidants that contribute to overall well-being and help prevent deficiencies.

While plant-based diets offer numerous health benefits, it's essential to plan meals carefully to ensure adequate intake of certain nutrients that may be less abundant or less bioavailable from plant sources alone. Key nutrients to pay attention to include vitamin B12, vitamin D, iron, calcium, omega-3 fatty acids, and protein. Fortified foods and supplements can be useful in meeting these needs, especially for those who follow strict vegan diets.

Transitioning to a plant-based diet can be gradual, allowing time to adjust tastes and learn new recipes. Experimenting with different foods and cooking methods can make the transition more enjoyable and sustainable in the long term.

Ultimately, whether for health, environmental, ethical reasons, or a combination thereof, plant-based diets offer a viable and beneficial dietary choice. By focusing on whole, plant-derived foods and ensuring balanced nutrition, individuals can thrive while reducing their carbon footprint and supporting sustainable food systems.

WHAT CONSTITUTES A PLANT-BASED DIET?

A plant-based diet revolves around consuming foods primarily sourced from plants, including fruits, vegetables, whole grains, legumes, nuts, seeds, and oils. This dietary approach places a strong emphasis on minimizing or altogether excluding animal products and heavily processed foods. The extent of restriction regarding animal products can vary widely depending on individual preferences and specific types of plant-based diets.

Central to a plant-based diet is the prioritization of whole, unrefined, or minimally processed plant foods. These foods are inherently rich in essential nutrients such as fiber, vitamins, minerals, and phytonutrients, which are beneficial for overall health and well-being. By focusing on plant-derived sources, individuals can naturally achieve a diet that supports a diverse array of nutritional needs.

Unlike strict vegetarian or vegan diets that completely exclude animal-derived foods, a plant-based diet offers flexibility. This flexibility allows individuals to adjust the degree of inclusion of animal products based on personal health goals, ethical considerations, or cultural factors. Some may choose to occasionally include small amounts of dairy, eggs, or lean meats, while others may opt for a more stringent avoidance of all animal products.

The versatility of a plant-based diet makes it accessible to a wide range of people, accommodating various dietary preferences and requirements. Whether someone is aiming to improve cardiovascular health, manage weight, or reduce their environmental footprint, adopting a plant-based diet can align with these goals. Furthermore, the emphasis on whole foods encourages mindful eating practices, promoting long-term health benefits beyond just nutritional intake.

In essence, a plant-based diet is characterized by its foundation in plant-derived foods, offering a nutritious and adaptable approach to eating that can be tailored to suit individual lifestyles and health objectives. By prioritizing natural, nutrient-dense foods and minimizing reliance on processed items and animal products, individuals can cultivate a balanced and sustainable dietary pattern that supports overall health and well-being.

TYPES OF PLANT-BASED DIETS

1. Vegan Diet: The vegan diet is the most restrictive among plant-based diets,

excluding all animal products. This includes meat, poultry, fish, dairy, eggs, and even honey. Vegans rely exclusively on plant-derived foods for their nutritional needs. This dietary choice often extends beyond food consumption to exclude any products derived from animals, such as leather or wool.

2. Vegetarian Diet: Vegetarian diets exclude meat, poultry, and fish, but they may include other animal-derived products depending on the type:

a.   Lacto-vegetarian: Includes dairy products but excludes eggs.

b.   Ovo-vegetarian: Includes eggs but excludes dairy products.

c.   Lacto-ovo vegetarian: Includes both dairy products and eggs. This is the most common type of vegetarian diet and allows for a broader range of food choices compared to strict veganism.

3. Flexitarian Diet: Also known as semi-vegetarianism, the flexitarian diet is more flexible compared to other plant-based diets. It primarily consists of plant-based foods but allows for occasional consumption of meat, poultry, fish, or dairy products. The emphasis remains on plant foods, with the inclusion of animal products in moderation. This flexibility makes it easier for individuals to transition towards a predominantly plant-based diet without completely eliminating animal products.

Each type of plant-based diet offers unique benefits. Vegan diets, for example, are typically higher in fiber, antioxidants, and certain vitamins, while vegetarian diets that include dairy and eggs can provide additional protein and essential nutrients like calcium and vitamin B12. Flexitarian diets provide a middle ground, offering the health benefits associated with plant-based diets while allowing occasional flexibility for personal or social reasons.

NUTRITIONAL BENEFITS OF A PLANT-BASED DIET

Plant-based diets are celebrated for their manifold nutritional advantages, particularly in bolstering overall health and potentially alleviating symptoms for

those grappling with autoimmune disorders.

Firstly, plant-based diets are inherently abundant in essential nutrients vital for bodily functions. They boast a diverse array of vitamins such as vitamin C, known for its immune-boosting properties, vitamin A crucial for vision and skin health, and folate, essential for cell division and growth. Additionally, minerals like potassium, magnesium, and calcium are plentiful, supporting various physiological processes from muscle function to bone health. These nutrients collectively fortify the immune system, mitigate inflammation, and foster general well-being.

Another hallmark of plant-based diets is their high fiber content. Fiber plays a pivotal role in digestive health by promoting regular bowel movements and preventing constipation. Moreover, it aids in regulating blood sugar levels, which is particularly beneficial in managing conditions like diabetes. Additionally, fiber contributes to a sense of satiety, aiding in weight management. Furthermore, fiber acts as a prebiotic, nourishing the beneficial bacteria in the gut microbiota. A healthy gut microbiota, in turn, bolsters immune function and modulates inflammation, crucial for individuals grappling with autoimmune ailments.

Compared to animal-based diets, plant-based diets tend to be lower in saturated fats and cholesterol. Elevated levels of saturated fats are linked to increased inflammation and a heightened risk of cardiovascular ailments, often interconnected with autoimmune conditions. By minimizing saturated fats and cholesterol, plant-based diets offer a pathway to reduce inflammation and bolster heart health.

Moreover, plant foods are replete with antioxidants, such as flavonoids and carotenoids, which shield cells from oxidative stress induced by free radicals. Antioxidants confer protective benefits, potentially curbing inflammation and reinforcing immune resilience. This antioxidant-rich profile underscores the therapeutic potential of plant-based diets in managing autoimmune disorders.

Certain components of plant-based diets exhibit anti-inflammatory properties as well. Omega-3 fatty acids found in walnuts and flaxseeds, and phytochemicals abundant in colorful fruits and vegetables, exert anti-inflammatory effects. These bioactive compounds mitigate inflammation, potentially alleviating symptoms associated with autoimmune diseases.

CHAPTER FOUR

PLANT-BASED DIETS AND INFLAMMATION

Plant-based diets have gained attention for their potential to reduce inflammation in the body. Inflammation is a natural immune response, but chronic inflammation can contribute to various diseases like heart disease, diabetes, and arthritis. Here's how plant-based diets may help:

Firstly, plant-based diets are rich in anti-inflammatory compounds such as antioxidants, phytochemicals, and fiber. Fruits and vegetables, staples of plant-based eating, are packed with vitamins (like vitamin C and E) and minerals (such as magnesium and zinc) that combat oxidative stress and inflammation.

Secondly, plant-based diets are typically low in pro-inflammatory foods. Animal products like red meat and processed meats contain high levels of saturated fats and advanced glycation end products (AGEs), which can trigger inflammation when consumed in excess. By reducing or eliminating these foods, plant-based diets may help lower chronic inflammation markers.

Moreover, plant-based diets promote a healthy gut microbiome. A diverse array of plant foods provides prebiotics—fiber sources that feed beneficial gut bacteria. These bacteria produce short-chain fatty acids like butyrate, which have anti-inflammatory effects throughout the body.

Studies support the anti-inflammatory benefits of plant-based diets. Research has shown that individuals following vegetarian or vegan diets often have lower levels of inflammatory markers such as C-reactive protein (CRP) and interleukin-6 (IL-6) compared to omnivores. This suggests that plant-based diets may mitigate systemic inflammation.

Additionally, plant-based diets are associated with a lower risk of chronic diseases linked to inflammation. For instance, populations with higher plant food intake tend to have lower rates of cardiovascular disease, type 2 diabetes, and certain cancers—all conditions influenced by chronic inflammation. However, it's essential to note that not all plant-based diets are inherently anti-inflammatory. Highly processed plant-based foods like sugary snacks or refined grains can still contribute to inflammation. A balanced plant-based diet emphasizing whole foods like fruits, vegetables, whole grains, nuts, seeds, and legumes is key to reaping anti-inflammatory benefits.

HOW PLANT-BASED DIETS REDUCE INFLAMMATION

Plant-based diets are renowned for their ability to combat inflammation through a variety of nutritional mechanisms. By focusing on whole, unprocessed plant foods, these diets naturally incorporate numerous anti-inflammatory compounds essential for maintaining health.

Firstly, plant-based diets are rich in foods known for their anti-inflammatory properties. This includes a diverse array of fruits, vegetables, whole grains, legumes, nuts, seeds, and healthy oils like olive oil. These foods contain vitamins, minerals, and phytonutrients that actively reduce inflammation and support overall immune function.

A key component of plant foods is their high fiber content, which plays a crucial role in inflammation reduction. Dietary fiber promotes the growth of beneficial gut bacteria, leading to the production of short-chain fatty acids (SCFAs). SCFAs help regulate the immune system and decrease inflammation throughout the body.

Healthy fats are also integral to plant-based eating patterns. Sources such as nuts, seeds, avocados, and olive oil provide monounsaturated and polyunsaturated fats, including omega-3 fatty acids. These fats possess potent anti-inflammatory properties, contributing to the overall anti-inflammatory effect of plant-based diets.

Moreover, plant foods are abundant in phytonutrients such as flavonoids, carotenoids, and polyphenols. These compounds act as antioxidants, scavenging free radicals and reducing oxidative stress. By doing so, they mitigate inflammation and support cellular health, thereby lowering the risk of chronic inflammatory conditions.

In contrast to diets high in animal products, plant-based diets inherently reduce the intake of pro-inflammatory foods. Red and processed meats, saturated fats, and refined sugars, common in Western diets, are minimized or excluded in plant-based eating. By avoiding these inflammatory triggers, individuals can significantly decrease systemic inflammation levels.

Overall, the holistic approach of plant-based diets to inflammation reduction is multifaceted and scientifically supported. By incorporating a variety of anti-inflammatory foods, promoting beneficial gut bacteria through fiber intake, emphasizing healthy fats, harnessing the power of phytonutrients, and reducing pro-inflammatory food sources, these diets offer a comprehensive strategy for improving overall health and well-being. Adopting a plant-based diet not only supports individual health goals but also contributes to a sustainable and environmentally friendly food system.

KEY ANTI-INFLAMMATORY NUTRIENTS IN PLANT FOODS

Plant-based foods offer a wealth of nutrients renowned for their potent anti-inflammatory properties. Among these, omega-3 fatty acids stand out, particularly EPA and DHA found in flaxseeds, chia seeds, walnuts, and algae-based supplements. These fatty acids are crucial for reducing inflammation throughout the body.

Additionally, antioxidants play a pivotal role in combating inflammation by neutralizing harmful free radicals. Plant foods provide a rich array of antioxidants such as vitamin C, vitamin E, selenium, zinc, and phytochemicals like flavonoids and resveratrol. These compounds are abundant in fruits, vegetables, nuts, and seeds, contributing significantly to overall health and inflammation management.

Turmeric, renowned for its active compound curcumin, boasts remarkable anti-inflammatory and antioxidant effects. Studies highlight its potential in alleviating inflammation associated with autoimmune conditions, making it a valuable addition to anti-inflammatory diets.

Another notable anti-inflammatory agent found in plant foods is quercetin, a flavonoid present in apples, onions, and berries. Quercetin helps modulate inflammatory pathways and reduces oxidative stress, offering protective benefits against chronic inflammation. Polyphenols, widely present in green tea, red grapes, and dark chocolate, are celebrated for their anti-inflammatory properties. These compounds contribute to the overall health benefits associated with plant-based diets, supporting cardiovascular health and immune function while mitigating inflammation. Incorporating these nutrients into daily meals can have profound effects on reducing systemic inflammation and promoting overall well-being. Whether through omega-3 fatty acids from seeds and algae, antioxidants from colorful fruits and vegetables, curcumin-rich turmeric, quercetin-packed fruits and onions, or polyphenol-rich beverages and treats, plant-based sources offer a diverse arsenal against inflammatory processes.

By emphasizing a varied and balanced intake of these nutrients, individuals can proactively manage inflammation and support long-term health. Whether as part of a targeted dietary approach or a broader lifestyle shift towards plant-centric eating, these nutrients showcase nature's potent ability to nurture and heal the body from within, promoting vitality and resilience against inflammatory challenges.

CASE STUDIES AND RESEARCH FINDINGS

Research into the impact of plant-based diets on inflammation and autoimmune diseases has yielded promising findings across various conditions:

Rheumatoid Arthritis (RA): Studies suggest that adopting plant-based diets rich in fruits, vegetables, and whole grains may offer significant benefits for individuals with rheumatoid arthritis. These diets have shown potential in reducing inflammation markers and improving symptoms such as joint pain and stiffness. The emphasis on anti-inflammatory foods and nutrients may contribute to better disease management and quality of life for RA patients.

Multiple Sclerosis (MS): Preliminary research indicates that diets low in saturated fats and high in fruits, vegetables, and omega-3 fatty acids could potentially mitigate inflammation and slow disease progression in multiple sclerosis. While further investigation is warranted, these dietary patterns appear promising in supporting the immune system and nervous system health in MS patients.

Inflammatory Bowel Disease (IBD): Plant-based diets have shown promise in managing inflammation and symptoms associated with Crohn's disease and ulcerative colitis, the two main forms of IBD. Although responses vary among individuals, some studies suggest that diets emphasizing plant foods may help modulate immune responses and improve gut health, leading to reduced disease activity and improved well-being.

General Health Benefits: Beyond specific autoimmune conditions, adopting a plant-based diet has been linked to lower levels of inflammatory markers such as C-reactive protein (CRP) and interleukin-6 (IL-6). Population studies indicate that plant-based diets are associated with reduced risks of cardiovascular diseases, hypertension, and metabolic syndrome. The abundance of antioxidants, phytochemicals, fiber, and healthy fats in plant foods contributes to overall health improvements, including better weight management and lower incidence of chronic diseases.

Overall, the evidence supports the notion that plant-based diets can play a beneficial role in managing inflammation and autoimmune diseases. By focusing on nutrient-dense plant foods and minimizing processed foods and animal products, individuals may potentially alleviate symptoms, reduce inflammation, and enhance their overall health outcomes. Further research, including long-term studies and randomized controlled trials, is essential to fully understand the mechanisms and optimize dietary recommendations for autoimmune disease management.

CHAPTER FIVE

ESSENTIAL NUTRIENTS IN A PLANT-BASED DIET

A plant-based diet offers a wealth of essential nutrients crucial for overall health and well-being. While it primarily revolves around fruits, vegetables, grains, legumes, nuts, and seeds, understanding which nutrients are key can help ensure a balanced intake.

Protein: Contrary to popular belief, plant-based diets can provide abundant protein. Legumes like beans, lentils, and chickpeas, as well as tofu and tempeh, are excellent sources. Whole grains such as quinoa and bulgur also contribute protein.

Fiber: Found abundantly in plants, fiber aids digestion, promotes satiety, and supports heart health. Fruits, vegetables, whole grains, nuts, and seeds are rich sources.

Vitamins and Minerals:

a. Vitamin C: Crucial for immune function and skin health, found in citrus fruits, strawberries, bell peppers, and broccoli.

b. Vitamin A: Essential for vision and immune function, abundant in carrots, sweet potatoes, and leafy greens.

c. Vitamin K: Important for blood clotting and bone health, found in spinach, kale, and broccoli.

d. Folate (Vitamin B9): Vital for cell division and red blood cell formation, found in leafy greens, beans, and fortified grains.

e. Iron: Necessary for oxygen transport, prevalent in lentils, beans, tofu, and spinach. Consuming vitamin C-rich foods enhances iron absorption.

f. Calcium: Critical for bone health and muscle function, found in fortified plant milks, tofu, kale, and almonds.

g. Iodine: Essential for thyroid function, seaweed and iodized salt are good sources.

h. Zinc: Supports immune function and metabolism, found in beans, lentils, and seeds.

Omega-3 Fatty Acids: Vital for heart and brain health, plant sources include flaxseeds, chia seeds, walnuts, and hemp seeds.

Antioxidants: Protect cells from damage, found abundantly in berries, leafy greens, and nuts.

Phytonutrients: Plant compounds with health-promoting properties, such as flavonoids in berries and quercetin in apples, contribute to overall well-being.

Challenges and Considerations: While plant-based diets offer numerous benefits, attention to certain nutrients like vitamin B12 (found in fortified foods or supplements), vitamin D (sunlight exposure or supplements), and ensuring adequate protein intake are essential.

Balanced Approach: Incorporating a variety of foods ensures a diverse nutrient intake. Whole grains, legumes, nuts, seeds, fruits, and vegetables provide complementary nutrients that support overall health.

MACRONUTRIENTS: PROTEIN, CARBOHYDRATES, FATS

Macronutrients are essential components of a balanced diet, comprising protein, carbohydrates, and fats. In a plant-based diet, protein sources are diverse and include beans such as chickpeas, black beans, and lentils, as well as soy-based products like tofu and tempeh. Other options like edamame, quinoa, nuts such as almonds and walnuts, seeds like chia and hemp seeds, and whole grains including oats and brown rice also provide significant protein content. To ensure adequate intake of all essential amino acids, combining different plant protein sources throughout the day is recommended.

Carbohydrates in plant-based diets predominantly consist of complex carbohydrates sourced from fruits, vegetables, and whole grains like barley, quinoa, and whole wheat. Legumes such as beans and lentils, along with starchy vegetables like potatoes and sweet potatoes, are also rich sources of carbohydrates. These complex carbohydrates not only supply energy but also deliver fiber, vitamins, and minerals crucial for overall health and wellbeing.

Healthy fats play a vital role in plant-based nutrition, sourced primarily from avocados, nuts such as almonds, walnuts, and cashews, seeds like flaxseeds and chia seeds, and oils including olive oil and coconut oil. These fats are rich in essential fatty acids like omega-3 and omega-6, which are fundamental for supporting brain health, hormone production, and overall cellular function.

MICRONUTRIENTS: VITAMINS AND MINERALS

Micronutrients are essential components of a balanced diet, encompassing vitamins and minerals crucial for maintaining overall health and well-being. Plant-based foods are rich sources of these micronutrients, offering a wide array of vitamins and minerals vital for various bodily functions.

Vitamins play diverse roles in the body, and plant-based sources abound with these nutrients: Vitamin A, pivotal for vision and immune function, is plentiful in orange and yellow fruits like carrots and sweet potatoes, as well as in leafy greens such as spinach and kale. Vitamin C, renowned for its antioxidant properties and role in immune health, can be found abundantly in citrus fruits like oranges and lemons, as well as in strawberries, bell peppers, and broccoli. Vitamin E, crucial for skin health and as an antioxidant, is present in nuts such as almonds and sunflower seeds, seeds like hazelnuts and pumpkin seeds, and vegetable oils. B Vitamins, a complex of essential nutrients vital for energy metabolism and nerve function, are abundant in whole grains such as brown rice and oats, legumes like lentils and beans, leafy greens, and fortified plant-based milk such as almond or soy milk.

Minerals are equally vital, supporting various physiological functions: Iron, critical for oxygen transport and found abundantly in plant-based sources like beans, lentils, tofu, spinach, quinoa, and fortified cereals. Calcium, essential for bone health and muscle function, is prevalent in leafy greens like kale and collard greens, fortified plant-based milk, calcium-set tofu, almonds, and sesame seeds. Zinc, crucial for immune function and wound healing, is found in legumes such as chickpeas and lentils, nuts like cashews and almonds, seeds such as pumpkin seeds, and whole grains. Magnesium, important for muscle and nerve function, is abundant in nuts such as almonds and cashews, seeds like sunflower and flaxseeds, leafy greens, whole grains, and legumes. Incorporating a variety of these plant-based foods into one's diet ensures an adequate intake of vitamins and minerals essential for optimal health. Whether through colorful fruits and vegetables, nutrient-dense nuts and seeds, or wholesome grains and legumes, plant-based diets offer a wealth of micronutrients necessary for supporting overall wellness and vitality.

SOURCES OF ESSENTIAL NUTRIENTS IN PLANT-BASED FOODS

Plant-based diets are renowned for their rich variety of foods that supply essential nutrients vital for overall health and well-being. By incorporating a diverse array of plant-based sources, individuals can easily meet their nutritional needs across various categories.

Protein is a critical component in any diet, and plant-based options abound. Legumes such as beans and lentils offer substantial protein content, complemented by soy-based products like tofu and tempeh. Nuts and seeds, such as almonds, walnuts, chia seeds, and flaxseeds, contribute not only protein but also healthy fats and essential minerals. Quinoa, a versatile pseudo-grain, and various whole grains like oats and brown rice are additional protein sources that enhance dietary diversity.

Carbohydrates, essential for energy, are plentiful in plant-based diets. Fruits and vegetables form the foundation, providing a spectrum of complex carbohydrates along with fiber and essential vitamins. Whole grains such as oats and brown rice offer sustained energy release, while legumes like beans and lentils provide a hearty carbohydrate source alongside their protein content. Starchy vegetables like sweet potatoes and squash round out the carbohydrate profile, offering both sustenance and essential nutrients.

Fats, another crucial macronutrient, are well-represented in plant-based foods. Avocados are a nutrient-dense source of healthy monounsaturated fats, while nuts and seeds contribute polyunsaturated fats and omega-3 fatty acids crucial for heart health. Plant oils, including olive oil and coconut oil, are versatile additions that provide both flavor and essential fatty acids necessary for bodily functions.

Vitamins and minerals are abundant in plant-based diets, primarily sourced from leafy green vegetables and colorful fruits and vegetables. These foods are rich in vitamins A, C, and K, as well as various B vitamins essential for metabolism and overall health. Nuts, seeds, and whole grains provide minerals such as magnesium, zinc, and iron, crucial for immune function and oxygen transport in the body. Fortified plant-based products, including alternative milks and cereals, offer additional sources of calcium, vitamin D, and vitamin B12, which are typically lower in plant-based diets.

CHAPTER SIX

PLANNING A BALANCED PLANT-BASED DIET FOR AUTOIMMUNE HEALTH

1. Focus on Variety:

Incorporate a wide range of fruits, vegetables, whole grains, legumes, nuts, and seeds. This ensures you get a diverse array of nutrients, including essential vitamins, minerals, and antioxidants, which are crucial for managing inflammation and supporting immune function.

2. Prioritize Anti-Inflammatory Foods:

Some plant-based foods are particularly known for their anti-inflammatory properties. These include:

a.   Berries: Blueberries, strawberries, and raspberries are rich in antioxidants.

b.   Leafy Greens: Spinach, kale, and Swiss chard provide essential nutrients and antioxidants.

c.   Cruciferous Vegetables: Broccoli, cauliflower, and Brussels sprouts contain compounds that reduce inflammation.

d.   Nuts and Seeds: Flaxseeds, chia seeds, and walnuts are high in omega-3 fatty acids.

3. Ensure Adequate Protein Intake:
Plant-based proteins are essential for repair and maintenance of body tissues. Include:

a.   Legumes: Beans, lentils, and chickpeas are excellent protein sources.

b.   Soy Products: Tofu, tempeh, and edamame offer high-quality protein.

c. Nuts and Seeds: Almonds, sunflower seeds, and hemp seeds also contribute protein.

4. Healthy Fats:

Healthy fats are crucial for reducing inflammation. Focus on:

a.   Avocado: A great source of healthy monounsaturated fats.

b.   Olive Oil: Use extra-virgin olive oil for cooking and dressings.

c.   Nuts and Seeds: As mentioned, these also provide healthy fats.

5. Whole Grains:

Whole grains provide fiber, B vitamins, and other nutrients. Choose:

a.   Quinoa: A complete protein source with all essential amino acids.

b.   Brown Rice: A versatile whole grain.

c.   Oats: Great for breakfast and baking.

6. Limit Processed Foods and Sugars:

Minimize intake of processed foods, which can exacerbate inflammation. Avoid sugary snacks, sodas, and refined grains.

7. Hydration:

Stay hydrated with plenty of water. Herbal teas can also be beneficial, particularly those with anti-inflammatory properties like turmeric and ginger tea.

8. Supplement Wisely:

Sometimes, certain nutrients may be challenging to obtain solely from a plant-based diet. Consider supplements for:

a.   Vitamin B12: Essential for nerve function and red blood cell production.

b.   Vitamin D: Important for immune health; consider a supplement, especially in low-sunlight months.

c.   Omega-3 Fatty Acids: If not getting enough from seeds and nuts, consider an algae-based supplement.

9. Listen to Your Body:

Monitor how different foods affect your symptoms. Some people with autoimmune conditions may find relief by avoiding gluten or nightshade vegetables (tomatoes, peppers, eggplants).

10. Consult a Healthcare Professional:

Before making significant dietary changes, consult with a healthcare provider or a registered dietitian, especially if you have specific health concerns or are on medication.

MEAL PLANNING AND PREPARATION

Weekly Meal Planning and Preparation Guide

1. Create a Weekly Meal Plan: Begin by outlining your meals for the entire week. Incorporate a variety of fruits, vegetables, whole grains, legumes, nuts, and seeds into your plan. This approach ensures you have all the necessary ingredients on hand, helping to minimize the temptation to opt for unhealthy food choices.

2. Batch Cooking: Engage in batch cooking to prepare large quantities of staple foods such as grains, beans, and roasted vegetables. These can be used in various meals throughout the week, saving time and guaranteeing that you always have nutritious options readily available.

3. Diverse Ingredients: Ensure your diet includes a wide range of plant-based foods to provide a broad spectrum of nutrients. Different colors of fruits and vegetables deliver various vitamins and antioxidants, essential for maintaining a balanced diet. For example, incorporating leafy greens, berries, carrots, and tomatoes can offer a rich mix of nutrients.

4. Simple Recipes: Opt for simple recipes that are both enjoyable and quick to prepare. This makes it easier to adhere to your dietary goals. Salads, stir-fries, soups, and grain bowls are versatile choices that can be customized with different ingredients to keep meals interesting and nutritious.

5. Healthy Snacks: Maintain a stock of healthy snacks such as fresh fruit, nuts, seeds, and hummus paired with vegetables. Having these options on hand helps prevent reaching for processed, unhealthy snacks when hunger strikes.

Practical Tips for Meal Planning

1. Preparation: Dedicate some time each week to plan and prepare your

meals. This might involve setting aside a few hours on a weekend to cook and store meals for the upcoming week.

2.   Storage: Invest in good quality storage containers to keep your batch-cooked meals fresh. Label them with dates to keep track of their shelf life.

3.   Variety: Rotate different recipes and ingredients weekly to keep your meals exciting and to ensure a varied intake of nutrients. For instance, try a different grain each week, such as quinoa, brown rice, or barley.

4.   Portion Control: Pre-portion your meals and snacks to avoid overeating and to make it easier to grab a healthy option on the go.

BALANCING MACRONUTRIENTS AND MICRONUTRIENTS

Balancing macronutrients and micronutrients is essential for maintaining optimal health and well-being. Here's how to ensure you're getting the right nutrients from your diet:

Macronutrients:

1. Protein: It's crucial to include a source of protein in every meal to support muscle repair and growth, as well as overall body function. Excellent plant-based protein options include beans, lentils, tofu, tempeh, nuts, seeds, and whole grains. These sources not only provide protein but also come with additional nutrients such as fiber and essential amino acids.

2.   Carbohydrates: Prioritize complex carbohydrates, which provide sustained energy and essential nutrients. Whole grains such as brown rice, quinoa, and oats, as well as starchy vegetables like sweet potatoes and legumes, are ideal choices. These foods have a low glycemic index, meaning they release energy slowly and help maintain stable blood sugar levels.

3.   Fats: Healthy fats are vital for brain health, hormone production, and overall cellular function. Include sources of unsaturated fats such as avocados, nuts, seeds, and plant oils like olive oil in your diet. These fats help reduce inflammation and support heart health.

Micronutrients:

1.   Vitamins: Consuming a variety of colorful fruits and vegetables ensures you get a broad spectrum of vitamins essential for various bodily functions. For instance, vitamin C, found in oranges, strawberries, and bell peppers, is crucial for immune function and skin health. Vitamin A, present in carrots, sweet potatoes, and leafy greens, supports vision, immune function, and cellular communication.

2.   Minerals: Adequate intake of minerals is necessary for bone health, oxygen transport, and enzyme function. Leafy greens like spinach and kale provide calcium and iron, essential for bone health and oxygen transport,

respectively. Nuts and seeds are excellent sources of magnesium, which supports muscle and nerve function, and zinc, which is vital for immune function and DNA synthesis. Whole grains also contribute to the intake of these and other minerals, making them a valuable component of a balanced diet.

TIPS FOR ENSURING ADEQUATE PROTEIN AND OTHER KEY NUTRIENTS

Ensuring adequate intake of protein and other essential nutrients is crucial, especially for those following a plant-based diet. Here are some detailed tips to help you maintain balanced nutrition:

Protein:

1. Combine Sources: To obtain all essential amino acids, it's beneficial to

mix different plant-based protein sources throughout the day. For example, you can have lentils at lunch and quinoa at dinner. This combination ensures that your body gets a complete protein profile.

2.   Protein-Rich Snacks: Incorporating snacks that are high in protein can help boost your overall intake. Nuts, seeds, and hummus are excellent options that are easy to include between meals.

Iron:

1.   Plant Sources: Include iron-rich foods such as lentils, chickpeas, spinach, and fortified cereals in your diet. These foods can help maintain healthy iron levels.

2.   Enhance Absorption: Iron from plant sources is not as easily absorbed by the body as iron from animal sources. Pairing iron-rich foods with vitamin C sources, like citrus fruits or bell peppers, can significantly enhance absorption. For example, having a spinach salad with lemon juice dressing can improve iron uptake.

Calcium:

1.   Plant Sources: Consume calcium-rich foods such as fortified plant-based milk, tofu made with calcium sulfate, almonds, and leafy greens. These foods can help meet your calcium needs without dairy.

2.   Consistent Intake: It's important to get calcium from multiple sources

throughout the day to ensure consistent levels in the body. Incorporate a variety of calcium-rich foods in your meals and snacks.

Vitamin B12:

1.	Supplementation: Vitamin B12 is not naturally present in plant foods. Consider taking a B12 supplement or consuming fortified foods like plant-based milk and nutritional yeast. These fortified foods can help maintain adequate B12 levels and prevent deficiencies.

Omega-3 Fatty Acids:

1.	Plant Sources: Include sources of alpha-linolenic acid (ALA) such as flaxseeds, chia seeds, walnuts, and hemp seeds in your diet. These foods provide essential fatty acids that support heart and brain health.

2. Algae-Based Supplements: For direct sources of DHA and EPA, which are more readily used by the body, consider algae-based supplements. These are particularly useful for those who do not consume fish.

Vitamin D:

1. Sun Exposure: Spending time outdoors helps the body produce vitamin D naturally. Aim for at least 10-30 minutes of midday sun exposure several times a week, depending on your skin type and location.

2. Supplementation: During the winter months or if you have limited sun exposure, taking a vitamin D

supplement can help maintain optimal levels. This is especially important in regions with long winters or for individuals with indoor lifestyles.

CHAPTER SEVEN

SUPERFOODS AND SUPPLEMENTS FOR AUTOIMMUNE SUPPORT

Managing autoimmune conditions can be challenging, but certain superfoods and supplements may help support the immune system and overall health. Here's a guide to some of the best options:

Superfoods for Autoimmune Support

1.   Leafy Greens:

a.   Examples: Spinach, kale, and Swiss chard.

b.   Benefits: Rich in vitamins A, C, and K, and minerals like iron and calcium, leafy greens help reduce inflammation and support immune function.

2.   Berries:

a.   Examples: Blueberries, strawberries, and raspberries.

b.   Benefits: High in antioxidants and vitamins, berries can help combat oxidative stress and inflammation, which are common in autoimmune conditions.

3.   Fatty Fish:

a.   Examples: Salmon, mackerel, and sardines.

b.   Benefits: Loaded with omega-3 fatty acids, these fish reduce inflammation and may help manage autoimmune symptoms.

4.   Nuts and Seeds:

a.   Examples: Walnuts, flaxseeds, and chia seeds.

b.   Benefits: Provide healthy fats, fiber, and antioxidants, which can help lower inflammation and support heart health.

5.   Cruciferous Vegetables:

a.   Examples: Broccoli, cauliflower, and Brussels sprouts.

b.   Benefits: Contain compounds that support detoxification and have anti-inflammatory properties.

6.   Turmeric:

a.   Benefits: Contains curcumin, a powerful anti-inflammatory compound that can help reduce symptoms of autoimmune conditions.

7.   Ginger:

a.   Benefits: Known for its anti-inflammatory and antioxidant effects, ginger can help alleviate pain and inflammation.

Supplements for Autoimmune Support

1. Vitamin D:

a. Benefits: Essential for immune function, vitamin D can help modulate the immune system and reduce autoimmune symptoms. Many people with autoimmune diseases are deficient in vitamin D.

2. Omega-3 Fatty Acids:

a. Sources: Fish oil supplements.

b. Benefits: These supplements can reduce inflammation and improve symptoms in conditions like rheumatoid arthritis.

3. Probiotics:

a.   Benefits: Support gut health, which is crucial for a balanced immune system. A healthy gut can help reduce the severity of autoimmune reactions.

4.   Magnesium:

a.   Benefits: Vital for many bodily functions, including muscle and nerve function, magnesium can help reduce symptoms like fatigue and muscle pain common in autoimmune diseases.

5.   Curcumin Supplements:

a.   Benefits: Concentrated curcumin can provide powerful anti-inflammatory effects, potentially reducing symptoms in autoimmune conditions.

6.   Glutathione:

a.   Benefits: A potent antioxidant that helps protect cells from damage, supports detoxification, and can help manage autoimmune symptoms.

7.   B Vitamins:

a.   Examples: B6, B12, and folate.

b.   Benefits: Important for energy production and immune function, B vitamins can help reduce fatigue and support overall health.

Tips for Using Superfoods and Supplements

1.   Consult with a Healthcare Professional: Before starting any new supplement, it's important to talk to a doctor, especially when dealing with autoimmune conditions.

2.   Balanced Diet: Focus on a well-rounded diet that includes a variety of nutrient-dense foods.

3.   Consistency: Regular consumption of these superfoods and supplements can help manage symptoms and support overall health.

4.   Monitor Reactions: Pay attention to how your body responds and adjust as necessary.

TOP ANTI-INFLAMMATORY SUPERFOODS

Turmeric: Renowned for its active compound curcumin, turmeric stands out for its potent anti-inflammatory and antioxidant properties. Curcumin can inhibit various molecules known to play major roles in inflammation. Incorporating turmeric into meals or enjoying a cup of turmeric tea can be an effective strategy to combat inflammation. For better absorption, pair it with black pepper or healthy fats.

Berries: Blueberries, strawberries, raspberries, and blackberries are among the top fruits for their rich content of antioxidants and vitamins. These berries help fight oxidative stress, a key factor in chronic inflammation. Their high levels of anthocyanins, quercetin, and vitamin C make them powerful anti-inflammatory agents. Regular consumption of these berries can significantly contribute to reducing inflammation and improving overall health.

Leafy Greens: Vegetables such as spinach, kale, and Swiss chard are loaded with essential vitamins, minerals, and antioxidants. These leafy greens are excellent sources of vitamin K, vitamin A, and folate, which support various bodily functions and reduce inflammatory markers. Including a variety of leafy greens in your diet can enhance your body's ability to fight inflammation and promote better health.

Nuts and Seeds: Almonds, walnuts, flaxseeds, and chia seeds are superb sources of healthy fats, fiber, and protein. These nuts and seeds are particularly rich in omega-3 fatty acids, which are known for their anti-inflammatory effects. Walnuts, for instance, contain alpha-linolenic acid (ALA), a type of omega-3 fatty acid that helps lower inflammation. Regularly consuming a mix of nuts and seeds can support heart health and reduce inflammation.

Fatty Fish: Salmon, mackerel, and sardines are packed with omega-3 fatty acids, specifically EPA and DHA, which have been extensively studied for their anti-inflammatory properties. These fatty acids help reduce the production of inflammatory compounds. For those following a plant-based diet, algae-based supplements can be a great alternative to obtain these essential fats. Incorporating fatty fish into your diet a few times a week can have significant anti-inflammatory benefits.

Ginger: This spice contains bioactive compounds such as gingerol, which possess strong anti-inflammatory and antioxidant effects. Ginger can help reduce inflammation and pain associated with conditions like osteoarthritis. Adding fresh ginger to your dishes or drinking ginger tea can be a delightful way to reap its benefits.

Green Tea: Known for its high polyphenol content, green tea is a potent anti-inflammatory beverage. The antioxidants in green tea, especially epigallocatechin gallate (EGCG), can help lower inflammation and protect against cellular damage. Regular consumption of green tea can support overall health and provide a soothing way to reduce inflammation.

SUPPLEMENTS TO CONSIDER

Many people, particularly those with autoimmune diseases, are deficient in vitamin D. This essential nutrient plays a crucial role in supporting immune function and reducing inflammation. Vitamin D supplements can help maintain adequate levels in the body, especially for individuals who have limited sun exposure or dietary intake of vitamin D-rich foods.

Vitamin B12 is another vital nutrient, essential for nerve health and the production of red blood cells. However, it is not naturally found in plant foods, making B12 supplements particularly important for those following a plant-based diet. Ensuring adequate intake of vitamin B12 can prevent deficiencies that lead to nerve damage and anemia, promoting overall health and wellbeing.

Omega-3 fatty acids, particularly EPA and DHA, are known for their anti-inflammatory properties and their ability to support heart and brain health. These fatty acids are typically found in fish oil or algae oil supplements. Regular consumption of omega-3 supplements can help reduce chronic inflammation, lower the risk of heart disease, and support cognitive function.

Probiotics are beneficial bacteria that support a healthy gut microbiome, which is essential for immune regulation. A balanced gut microbiome can help reduce inflammation and improve digestive health. Probiotic supplements can be particularly beneficial for individuals experiencing gastrointestinal issues or those who have been on antibiotics, which can disrupt the natural balance of gut bacteria.

Magnesium is a crucial mineral that supports muscle and nerve function, as well as immune health. Many people do not get enough magnesium from their diet, which can lead to deficiencies. Magnesium supplements can help maintain optimal levels of this mineral in the body, supporting various physiological functions and contributing to overall health.

Curcumin, the active compound found in turmeric, is renowned for its powerful anti-inflammatory properties. For those who cannot consume sufficient turmeric in their diet, curcumin supplements offer a concentrated source of this beneficial compound. Regular intake of curcumin can help manage inflammation and support joint and cardiovascular health.

HERBAL REMEDIES AND THEIR BENEFITS

Herbal remedies have been utilized for centuries across various cultures for their therapeutic properties, offering natural alternatives to support health and well-being. Here's a closer look at some prominent herbs and their benefits:

Echinacea: Celebrated for its immune-boosting capabilities, echinacea is renowned for reducing the frequency and severity of colds and infections. Its efficacy lies in stimulating the immune system, making it more robust against pathogens. Additionally, echinacea exhibits anti-inflammatory properties, aiding in the alleviation of symptoms associated with inflammation.

Boswellia: Commonly referred to as Indian frankincense, boswellia is revered for its potent anti-inflammatory effects. It has been traditionally used to manage conditions such as rheumatoid arthritis and inflammatory bowel disease, offering relief by reducing inflammation and associated discomfort.

Ashwagandha: As an adaptogenic herb, ashwagandha plays a pivotal role in helping the body cope with stress. By modulating the body's stress response, it supports overall immune function and contributes to reducing inflammation. Its adaptogenic properties make it a versatile remedy for promoting resilience and vitality.

Aloe Vera: Known for its soothing qualities, aloe vera is not just a topical remedy but also consumed as a juice for internal health benefits. It aids in reducing inflammation and supports digestive health, making it beneficial for conditions such as gastritis and irritable bowel syndrome.

Ginseng: Ginseng is prized for its anti-inflammatory and immune-boosting properties. It assists in reducing fatigue and enhancing overall well-being by supporting the immune system. Ginseng's adaptogenic nature also aids in mitigating stress effects on the body.

Milk Thistle: Recognized for its role in promoting liver health, milk thistle offers antioxidant and anti-inflammatory effects. It helps in detoxifying the body from harmful substances and supports liver function, making it particularly valuable for those with liver conditions or seeking to enhance detoxification processes.

Each of these herbs contributes uniquely to holistic health practices, offering natural alternatives that complement conventional treatments. Their benefits extend beyond mere symptom relief to enhancing the body's resilience and fostering overall vitality. Integrating these herbal remedies into a balanced lifestyle can provide substantial support for immune function, inflammation management, stress resilience, and organ health. As always, consulting with a healthcare provider is advisable before incorporating new herbs into your wellness regimen, especially if you have

existing health concerns or are taking
medications.

CHAPTER EIGHT

PRACTICAL TIPS FOR TRANSITIONING TO A PLANT-BASED DIET

1. Take it Slow: Start by gradually replacing one or two meals a day with plant-based options. This allows your taste buds and digestion to adjust gradually.

2. Explore New Foods: Experiment with a variety of fruits, vegetables, grains, legumes, nuts, and seeds. Try different recipes and cooking methods to find what you enjoy.

3. Plan Balanced Meals: Ensure your meals are balanced with a mix of carbohydrates, proteins, healthy fats, vitamins, and minerals. Include sources

of protein like beans, lentils, tofu, or tempeh.

4.   Read Labels: Learn to read food labels to identify hidden animal products like dairy derivatives and gelatin. Many packaged foods contain these ingredients.

5.   Stock Your Kitchen: Keep your pantry stocked with plant-based staples like whole grains (quinoa, brown rice), canned beans, nuts, seeds, and plant-based milk alternatives.

6.   Find Substitutes: Discover plant-based alternatives for your favorite animal-based foods. For example, use almond milk instead of cow's milk, or tofu instead of meat in stir-fries.

7.   Eat Out Mindfully: When dining out, research vegan-friendly restaurants or check the menu online beforehand. Many restaurants offer plant-based options or can modify dishes upon request.

8.   Join a Community: Connect with others who follow a plant-based diet for support and recipe ideas. Online forums, social media groups, and local meetups can be great resources.

9.   Focus on Whole Foods: Choose whole, unprocessed foods as much as possible. They are typically richer in nutrients and fiber compared to processed alternatives.

10. Stay Informed: Educate yourself about nutrition to ensure you're meeting

your dietary needs. Consider consulting a registered dietitian if you have specific health concerns or questions.

11.   Listen to Your Body: Pay attention to how your body responds to the changes. You may need to adjust your diet to ensure you're getting enough nutrients, especially vitamin B12, iron, and omega-3 fatty acids.

12. Be   Patient: Remember, transitioning to any new diet takes time. Be patient with yourself and celebrate your progress along the way.

GRADUAL TRANSITION STRATEGIES

Transitioning to a more plant-based diet can be a rewarding journey towards better health and sustainability. By adopting gradual strategies, you can make this shift smoothly and sustainably.

Start with Small Steps: Begin by integrating more plant-based meals into your weekly routine. A practical approach is to designate one day, such as "Meatless Monday," for plant-based meals. Over time, gradually increase the frequency of plant-based meals as you become more comfortable and familiar with new recipes and ingredients.

Focus on Whole Foods: Emphasizing whole, unprocessed plant foods forms the foundation of a nutritious plant-based diet. These foods include fruits, vegetables, whole grains, legumes, nuts, and seeds, which are rich in essential nutrients, fiber, and antioxidants. They not only support overall health but also provide sustained energy levels throughout the day.

Experiment with Recipes: Explore the vast array of plant-based recipes available in cookbooks, online resources, and social media platforms. Experiment with different cooking techniques and flavor profiles to discover delicious and satisfying plant-based meals that suit your taste preferences and nutritional needs.

Meal Prep: Dedicate a specific time each week to plan and prepare meals ahead. Batch cooking staples like grains, beans, and roasted vegetables can save time during busy weekdays. Having prepared ingredients on hand makes it easier to assemble nutritious meals quickly, reducing the temptation to opt for less healthy options.

Find Plant-Based Alternatives: Identify plant-based alternatives for your favorite dishes to make the transition more seamless. For example, use tofu or tempeh instead of meat in stir-fries or opt for cashew cream instead of dairy cream in sauces. These alternatives can provide similar textures and flavors while being lower in saturated fats and cholesterol.

Transitioning to a plant-based diet is not just about what you exclude but also about embracing a variety of nutrient-dense foods that support your well-being. By starting gradually, focusing on whole foods, experimenting with new recipes, preparing meals ahead, and finding suitable alternatives, you can successfully transition to a more plant-centered way of eating that is both enjoyable and sustainable in the long term.

OVERCOMING COMMON CHALLENGES

Transitioning to a plant-based diet presents several common challenges, each of which can be effectively managed with mindful planning and awareness.

Firstly, ensuring sufficient protein intake is key. Incorporate a variety of plant-based sources such as beans, lentils, tofu, tempeh, nuts, seeds, and quinoa into your meals. Combining different protein sources throughout the day ensures you receive all essential amino acids necessary for optimal health.

Meeting nutrient needs is another critical aspect. Pay attention to nutrients like vitamin B12, iron, calcium, omega-3 fatty acids, and vitamin D. Supplements or fortified foods can be beneficial, especially if your diet may lack these essential nutrients.

Navigating social pressures can be challenging. Informing friends and family about your dietary choices beforehand can ease tensions. When attending gatherings, offer to bring a plant-based dish or choose restaurants that offer suitable options, ensuring you stay true to your dietary preferences without feeling isolated.

Managing cravings and adjusting to new tastes are natural parts of the transition. Experiment with plant-based versions of your favorite meals to satisfy cravings while adapting to new flavors and textures over time.

Educating yourself about the nutritional benefits of plant-based eating is empowering. Understanding how it can positively impact health, including managing conditions like autoimmune disorders, can reinforce your commitment and motivation to maintain this dietary choice.

Eating out and navigating social situations as a plant-based eater can be enjoyable with a bit of preparation and flexibility. Here are some practical tips to make dining out and socializing easier:

Firstly, it's beneficial to research restaurants ahead of time. Look for places that either have dedicated plant-based menus or are known to be accommodating to dietary preferences. Many eateries now offer plant-based options due to increasing demand, so checking their menus online or calling ahead can save you time and ensure you have choices available.

When you arrive at the restaurant, communicate your dietary needs clearly to the waitstaff. Don't hesitate to ask questions about ingredients or request modifications to suit your plant-based preferences. Most restaurants are willing to accommodate such requests if communicated politely and clearly.

In situations where the restaurant's options are limited, it can be helpful to have a backup plan. Bringing along plant-based snacks like fresh fruit, nuts, or energy bars ensures you won't go hungry if suitable meal options aren't available. This is particularly handy for social gatherings or events where the food choices might not align with your dietary preferences.

Consider hosting gatherings at your home as another strategy. By preparing and serving delicious plant-based dishes, you can introduce friends and family to the variety and flavors of plant-based eating. This not only expands their culinary horizons but also ensures you have full control over the meal's ingredients and suitability.

Flexibility is key in navigating social situations where plant-based options may be limited. Focus on choosing dishes that are predominantly plant-based and find ways to complement them with other available foods. For example, you might opt for a salad or vegetable-based dish and supplement it with sides or appetizers that meet your dietary needs.

Overall, being prepared, communicating clearly, and maintaining flexibility are essential strategies for enjoying dining out and socializing as a plant-based eater. With more restaurants catering to diverse dietary preferences and an increasing awareness of plant-based eating, it's becoming easier to find satisfying options wherever you go. By taking these proactive steps, you can ensure that your dining experiences are enjoyable, social, and aligned with your personal dietary choices.

☐

CHAPTER NINE

MANAGING SPECIFIC AUTOIMMUNE DISEASES WITH A PLANT-BASED DIET

Managing specific autoimmune diseases with a plant-based diet can be both beneficial and challenging depending on the condition. Autoimmune diseases occur when the immune system mistakenly attacks healthy tissues in the body, leading to inflammation and tissue damage. While diet alone may not cure autoimmune diseases, it can play a significant role in managing symptoms and improving overall health.

For conditions like rheumatoid arthritis (RA), a plant-based diet rich in fruits, vegetables, whole grains, and legumes can help reduce inflammation. These foods are typically high in antioxidants and phytochemicals, which have anti-inflammatory properties. Avoiding processed foods, red meat, and dairy products may also alleviate symptoms for some individuals by reducing inflammation triggers.

Similarly, people with lupus often find that a plant-based diet can help manage symptoms such as joint pain, fatigue, and skin rashes. Incorporating foods like leafy greens, berries, nuts, and seeds can provide essential nutrients and antioxidants while minimizing potential triggers that could worsen inflammation.

In the case of multiple sclerosis (MS), some studies suggest that a plant-based diet may support neurological health by reducing inflammation in the central nervous system. Foods rich in omega-3 fatty acids, such as flaxseeds, walnuts, and chia seeds, may be particularly beneficial.

However, transitioning to a plant-based diet can be challenging for individuals with autoimmune diseases, especially if they have specific dietary restrictions or nutrient deficiencies. It's crucial for individuals to work closely with healthcare providers or registered dietitians to ensure they're meeting their nutritional needs while avoiding potential deficiencies that could exacerbate symptoms.

Supplements like vitamin B12, vitamin D, and omega-3 fatty acids may need to be considered, as these nutrients are commonly found in animal products. Careful planning is essential to maintain a balanced diet that supports overall health and manages symptoms effectively.

Additionally, lifestyle factors such as stress management, regular exercise, and adequate sleep also play significant roles in managing autoimmune diseases. A holistic approach that combines a plant-based diet with these lifestyle adjustments can contribute to better disease management and improved quality of life for individuals living with autoimmune conditions.

Rheumatoid Arthritis (RA)

Rheumatoid Arthritis (RA) is a chronic autoimmune disorder marked by inflammation and pain in the joints. Managing RA involves adopting a diet rich in anti-inflammatory properties to alleviate symptoms and enhance overall well-being.

Central to an anti-inflammatory approach is emphasizing plant-based foods. Fruits, vegetables, whole grains, nuts, seeds, and legumes form the cornerstone of this diet due to their high levels of antioxidants and phytochemicals. These compounds help combat inflammation throughout the body, including in the joints affected by RA. By incorporating a variety of colorful fruits and vegetables, such as berries, leafy greens, and cruciferous vegetables, individuals can benefit from diverse anti-inflammatory properties.

Omega-3 fatty acids also play a crucial role in mitigating inflammation associated with RA. Sources like flaxseeds, chia seeds, walnuts, and algae-based supplements are rich in these beneficial fats. Omega-3s help modulate the immune response and support joint health, potentially reducing the severity of RA symptoms.

Conversely, minimizing intake of pro-inflammatory foods is equally important. Reducing or avoiding consumption of red meat, processed foods, and items high in saturated fats can help prevent exacerbation of inflammation. These dietary choices not only impact inflammation levels but also contribute to overall cardiovascular health and weight management, which are significant concerns for individuals with RA.

Research underscores the benefits of plant-based diets in managing RA symptoms. Studies suggest that such dietary patterns can lower inflammatory markers and improve outcomes such as joint pain and stiffness. This approach provides a holistic means of managing RA, complementing medical treatments and potentially reducing reliance on medications alone.

Multiple Sclerosis (MS) is a complex autoimmune disease that affects the central nervous system, causing a range of neurological symptoms. While its exact cause remains unclear, research suggests that lifestyle factors, including diet, may play a significant role in managing symptoms and promoting overall health in individuals with MS.

One dietary approach that has shown promise in supporting individuals with MS is a plant-based diet. This approach emphasizes whole plant foods such as fruits, vegetables, whole grains, nuts, seeds, and legumes, while minimizing or excluding animal products and processed foods.

Plant-based diets rich in omega-3 fatty acids have been highlighted for their potential to reduce inflammation, which is a key driver of MS progression. Omega-3s, found in abundance in sources like flaxseeds, chia seeds, walnuts, and certain algae, are known for their anti-inflammatory properties, which may help alleviate symptoms and support brain health in those with MS. Vitamin D also plays a crucial role in MS management, as the disease is associated with vitamin D deficiency. Adequate vitamin D levels can be maintained through safe sun exposure or supplements, which is important for regulating immune function and potentially reducing MS activity.

Additionally, whole plant foods are rich in essential nutrients, antioxidants, and fiber, which support overall health and may benefit individuals with MS by bolstering immune function and reducing oxidative stress.

Research into the specific benefits of plant-based diets for MS is ongoing but promising. Limited studies indicate that such diets may help reduce inflammation, improve overall quality of life, and potentially slow disease progression. However, more extensive research is needed to fully understand the impact and mechanisms of plant-based nutrition on MS outcomes.

Hashimoto's Thyroiditis is an autoimmune disorder that primarily affects the thyroid gland, resulting in hypothyroidism. Managing this condition through a plant-based diet involves strategic dietary choices aimed at supporting thyroid function and overall well-being.

Firstly, incorporating iodine-rich foods is crucial. Sources such as seaweed, iodized salt (in moderation), and certain nuts and seeds provide essential iodine necessary for thyroid hormone production. However, caution is advised with iodized salt due to its potential for excessive iodine intake, which can exacerbate thyroid issues.

Secondly, selenium plays a significant role in managing autoimmune thyroid conditions like Hashimoto's. Foods such as Brazil nuts, whole grains, and legumes are rich sources of selenium, which helps regulate thyroid function and reduce inflammation associated with autoimmune responses.

Additionally, some individuals with Hashimoto's may benefit from addressing gluten sensitivity. Gluten, found in grains like wheat, barley, and rye, can trigger autoimmune reactions in susceptible individuals, potentially worsening thyroid inflammation. Therefore, opting for gluten-free grains and avoiding processed foods containing gluten may alleviate symptoms for some patients.

Although specific studies linking plant-based diets directly to Hashimoto's management are limited, the diet's emphasis on nutrient-dense foods offers potential benefits. Plant-based diets typically include ample fruits, vegetables, whole grains, nuts, and seeds, which are rich in vitamins, minerals, antioxidants, and fiber. These nutrients support overall health and may indirectly contribute to thyroid function and immune system modulation.

It's important to note that individual responses to dietary changes can vary. Some individuals with Hashimoto's may find relief from symptoms by adopting a plant-based diet rich in whole, unprocessed foods. Others may need to customize their diet further, potentially incorporating additional dietary modifications or supplements under the guidance of a healthcare provider.

Lupus

Lupus is a complex autoimmune disease known for its systemic impact on various organs, joints, and tissues. Managing Lupus through a plant-based diet involves strategic dietary choices aimed at minimizing inflammation, supporting immune health, and enhancing overall well-being.

A cornerstone of the plant-based approach to managing Lupus is adopting an anti-inflammatory diet. This dietary pattern prioritizes fruits, vegetables, whole grains, and healthy fats such as those found in nuts, seeds, and olive oil. By focusing on these foods, individuals with Lupus can potentially reduce inflammation throughout the body, which is crucial as inflammation is a hallmark of autoimmune conditions like Lupus.

Omega-3 fatty acids play a significant role in managing inflammation and supporting heart health in Lupus patients. Sources of omega-3s include flaxseeds, chia seeds, walnuts, and fatty fish like salmon and mackerel. For those who prefer not to consume fish, plant-based supplements like algae-derived omega-3s offer a viable alternative to help manage symptoms associated with systemic inflammation.

Proper hydration is vital for individuals with Lupus, especially since the disease can affect kidney function. Water-rich fruits and vegetables such as cucumbers, strawberries, and celery not only contribute to hydration but also provide essential vitamins, minerals, and antioxidants that support overall health and immune function.

Research into the benefits of plant-based diets for Lupus management is promising. Studies suggest that such diets may help reduce inflammatory markers and alleviate symptoms such as fatigue and joint pain. By focusing on nutrient-dense plant foods, individuals with Lupus can potentially enhance their quality of life and better manage the chronic nature of the disease.

Other Conditions

Various autoimmune conditions, such as Psoriasis, Crohn's Disease, and Celiac Disease, can potentially benefit from adopting a plant-based diet tailored to specific needs and symptoms.

Psoriasis, characterized by skin inflammation and rapid cell turnover, often responds well to an anti-inflammatory diet. This approach involves emphasizing foods with anti-inflammatory properties, such as fruits, vegetables, nuts, and seeds. Avoiding trigger foods like processed sugars and dairy products that can exacerbate inflammation is crucial. By focusing on nutrient-dense plant-based options, individuals with psoriasis may experience reduced symptoms and improved skin health.

Crohn's Disease, a type of inflammatory bowel disease (IBD), affects the gastrointestinal tract. Managing this condition involves choosing foods that are gentle on the digestive system while promoting gut health and reducing inflammation. A plant-based diet rich in soluble fiber (found in oats, legumes, and fruits), easily digestible foods, and probiotics (from fermented foods like yogurt and sauerkraut) can help alleviate symptoms and support overall digestive function.

For those with Celiac Disease, an autoimmune disorder triggered by gluten, adopting a gluten-free plant-based diet is essential. This diet focuses on avoiding gluten-containing grains like wheat, barley, and rye, while incorporating naturally gluten-free whole foods such as quinoa, rice, fruits, vegetables, and legumes. This approach ensures individuals with Celiac Disease receive adequate nutrients and supports digestive healing by eliminating gluten, which can damage the small intestine in those with gluten sensitivity.

It's important to note that managing autoimmune conditions through diet requires a personalized approach. Individual factors such as specific symptoms, nutritional requirements, and food tolerances must be considered. Some individuals may find additional benefits from excluding other potential trigger foods or incorporating specific supplements to address deficiencies commonly associated with autoimmune diseases.

Overall, while a plant-based diet can offer significant benefits for autoimmune conditions like Psoriasis, Crohn's Disease, and Celiac Disease, consultation with healthcare professionals, such as registered dietitians or doctors specializing in autoimmune disorders, is advisable.

They can provide tailored dietary recommendations that align with individual health needs and optimize management of these complex conditions. By combining medical guidance with a well-planned plant-based diet, individuals can potentially reduce symptoms, support overall health, and improve their quality of life.

CHAPTER TEN

RECIPES AND MEAL PLANS

In this section, the focus is on supporting individuals who are transitioning to a plant-based diet, particularly for managing autoimmune conditions. It offers a variety of practical resources, including a diverse selection of recipes and sample meal plans.

The recipes provided cover breakfast, lunch, and dinner options, ensuring a comprehensive array of plant-based meals suitable for those with autoimmune concerns. Each recipe is crafted to not only meet nutritional needs but also to appeal to diverse tastes and preferences. Whether it's hearty breakfast ideas, satisfying lunch options, or flavorful dinner recipes, there's a variety to explore and enjoy.

Additionally, the section includes suggestions for snacks and smoothies. These ideas are designed to complement the main meals, offering nutritious and convenient choices for between-meal cravings or quick refreshments. Snack options are thoughtfully curated to provide energy boosts without compromising on healthfulness, making them ideal for those on the go or needing a quick bite.

To aid in practical implementation, a sample weekly meal plan is included. This plan serves as a blueprint for individuals looking to structure their week around balanced, plant-based meals. It not only helps beginners get started with the diet but also supports maintaining a healthy eating routine over time. The meal plan is designed to ensure a good balance of nutrients while accommodating the dietary needs often associated with autoimmune conditions. Overall, this section aims to empower individuals embarking on a plant-based diet journey with the tools they need to succeed. Whether seeking inspiration for a new breakfast routine, ideas for satisfying lunches, delicious dinner options, or simply guidance on how to structure their weekly eating habits, this resource provides comprehensive support. By combining practical recipes with a structured meal plan, it encourages a sustainable and balanced approach to plant-based eating tailored specifically for managing autoimmune health concerns.

BREAKFAST, LUNCH, AND DINNER RECIPES

For breakfast, kickstart your day with nutritious options like a Quinoa Breakfast Bowl. Simply cook quinoa and top it with a vibrant mix of fresh berries, nuts, seeds, and a touch of maple syrup for sweetness. Another quick and satisfying option is Avocado Toast: spread mashed avocado on whole grain toast and add cherry tomatoes and a sprinkle of nutritional yeast or hemp seeds for added flavor and nutrients. If you prefer something that can be prepared ahead, try Chia Seed Pudding: soak chia seeds in almond or coconut milk overnight, then in the morning, top with your favorite fruits and nuts for a refreshing and filling breakfast.

Moving on to lunch, aim for meals that are both filling and packed with nutrients. Consider a Mediterranean Chickpea Salad, where hearty chickpeas mingle with cucumbers, cherry tomatoes, olives, and red onion, all tossed in a zesty lemon-herb dressing. Alternatively, indulge in a Sweet Potato and Black Bean Burrito: fill a whole grain tortilla with roasted sweet potatoes, black beans, avocado slices, salsa, and leafy greens for a satisfying handheld meal. For a more substantial option, Quinoa-Stuffed Bell Peppers offer a colorful dish where bell peppers are stuffed with quinoa, mixed vegetables, and topped with marinara sauce and vegan cheese before baking.

As the day winds down, treat yourself to flavorful plant-based dinners. Try Stir-Fried Tofu with Vegetables, featuring tofu cubes stir-fried with bell peppers, broccoli, snap peas, and a ginger-garlic sauce, served over brown rice or noodles for a comforting meal. Another option is Lentil and Vegetable Curry, where red lentils simmer in coconut milk with tomatoes, spinach, and aromatic spices like turmeric, cumin, and coriander, perfect alongside quinoa or whole grain bread. For a satisfying burger alternative, indulge in Portobello Mushroom Burgers: grill marinated portobello mushroom caps in balsamic vinegar and olive oil, then serve on whole grain buns with lettuce, tomato, and creamy avocado.

These plant-based recipes not only cater to your nutritional needs but also offer a variety of flavors and textures to keep your meals exciting and enjoyable. Whether you're starting your day with a nutrient-packed breakfast, refueling at lunch with vibrant salads and burritos, or winding down with hearty dinners, these recipes provide delicious options to support your plant-based lifestyle.

SNACK AND SMOOTHIE IDEAS

Snacks and smoothies play a vital role in maintaining energy levels and providing essential nutrients throughout the day. Whether you're looking for a quick pick-me-up between meals or a refreshing beverage packed with goodness, here are some wholesome ideas to satisfy your cravings and nourish your body.

Healthy Snack Ideas

Fresh Fruit: Fresh fruits like apples, bananas, berries, and sliced oranges are not only delicious but also rich in vitamins, minerals, and fiber. They provide a natural sweetness and are easy to grab on the go or enjoy as a light snack at any time of the day.

Mixed Nuts and Seeds: Almonds, walnuts, pumpkin seeds, and sunflower seeds are excellent choices for a crunchy and satisfying snack. They are loaded with healthy fats, protein, and various micronutrients, offering a balance of energy and satiety.

Hummus and Veggies: Pairing hummus with fresh veggies such as carrot sticks, cucumber slices, and bell pepper strips creates a nutritious combination. Hummus provides protein and fiber, while vegetables offer vitamins, minerals, and hydration, making it a perfect snack for dipping.

Energy Bars: Whether homemade or store-bought, energy bars made with nuts, seeds, and dried fruits are convenient and provide a quick energy boost. They are often packed with antioxidants, healthy fats, and natural sugars, ideal for replenishing energy during busy days.

Nutrient-Packed Smoothie Ideas

Green Smoothie: A green smoothie is a fantastic way to incorporate leafy greens like spinach and kale into your diet, along with fruits and healthy fats. Blend together spinach, kale, banana, almond milk, and a spoonful of almond butter for a creamy and nutritious drink.

Berry Blast Smoothie: Berries such as strawberries, blueberries, and raspberries are loaded with antioxidants and vitamins. Combine them with plant-based yogurt, chia seeds for added fiber and omega-3s, and coconut water for hydration, creating a refreshing and vibrant smoothie.

Tropical Paradise Smoothie: For a taste of the tropics, blend pineapple, mango, spinach (for added greens), coconut milk for creaminess, and a squeeze of lime juice to brighten the flavors. This smoothie is not only delicious but also packed with vitamins, minerals, and healthy fats from coconut milk.

SAMPLE WEEKLY MEAL PLAN

Monday:

1.   Breakfast: Start the week with Overnight Oats made with almond milk, chia seeds, and sliced bananas. This fiber-rich and energizing dish prepares you for the day ahead.

2. Lunch: Enjoy a Mediterranean Chickpea Salad packed with fresh vegetables, olives, and a zesty dressing, providing a satisfying mix of protein and vitamins.

3. Dinner: Indulge in a hearty Lentil and Vegetable Curry served with quinoa, offering a complete protein source along with essential nutrients from a variety of vegetables.

Tuesday:

1. Breakfast: Treat yourself to Avocado Toast on whole grain bread, topped with a sprinkle of nutritional yeast or seeds for added crunch and nutrients.

2. Lunch: Savor a Sweet Potato and Black Bean Burrito, filled with fiber and

protein, complemented by your favorite salsa or guacamole.

3.   Dinner: Delight in Stir-Fried Tofu with a colorful array of vegetables over brown rice, providing a balanced meal with plenty of plant-based protein and complex carbohydrates.

Wednesday:

1.   Breakfast: Enjoy a refreshing Chia Seed Pudding topped with mixed berries, offering antioxidants, omega-3 fatty acids, and a delightful burst of flavor.

2.   Lunch: Relish Quinoa-Stuffed Bell Peppers, filled with quinoa, vegetables, and herbs, providing a wholesome and satisfying midday meal.

3. Dinner: Treat yourself to Portobello Mushroom Burgers served with a side salad, offering a savory and satisfying alternative to traditional burgers.

Thursday:

1. Breakfast: Blend a nutritious Smoothie with spinach, banana, almond milk, and almond butter, packed with vitamins, minerals, and healthy fats to fuel your morning.

2. Lunch: Enjoy leftover Lentil and Vegetable Curry for a quick and flavorful meal, reducing food waste while still enjoying a nutritious lunch.

3. Dinner: Have a flavorful Chickpea and Vegetable Stir-Fry with quinoa,

providing a protein-rich and vibrant dinner option.

Friday:

1.	Breakfast: Start your day with a Quinoa Breakfast Bowl topped with nuts and seeds for a crunchy texture and added protein, setting a nutritious tone for the weekend.

2.	Lunch: Wrap up the week with a Hummus and Veggie Wrap using a whole grain tortilla, filled with fresh vegetables and creamy hummus for a satisfying lunch.

3.	Dinner: Enjoy Cauliflower and Chickpea Curry served with brown rice, a comforting and nutrient-dense dish perfect for winding down the week.

Saturday:

1. Breakfast: Refresh with a Fruit Salad featuring assorted fruits and a sprinkle of nuts for added crunch and healthy fats.

2. Lunch: Dive into Tofu and Vegetable Stir-Fry over noodles, offering a delightful mix of flavors and textures for a satisfying midday meal.

3. Dinner: Enjoy a warming Eggplant and Tomato Stew served with couscous, providing a Mediterranean-inspired dish rich in antioxidants and flavors.

Sunday:

1. Breakfast: Blend a Smoothie with mixed berries, plant-based yogurt, and chia seeds, offering a refreshing and nutritious start to your Sunday morning.

2.   Lunch: Relish a Quinoa Salad with roasted vegetables and a lemon vinaigrette, providing a light yet satisfying meal to enjoy midday.

3.   Dinner: Wrap up the week with Spaghetti topped with Marinara Sauce and a side of steamed broccoli, a classic and comforting dinner option.

THE END